The Inflammation Advisor Series

INFLAMMATION 101

Natural Solutions
Beyond the Anti Inflammatory
Diet

Iris R. Bell, MD PhD

Disclaimer

The information provided here offers an educational resource only and is not intended to serve as nutritional, dietary, health, or medical advice related to any person's specific diet or health problems.

There can be no assurance that any person's specific diet or health problems, diseases, or symptoms will heal, recover, or otherwise resolve as a result of applying the information provided here or in other resources mentioned in the book.

There also can be no assurance of safety with or absence of possible harm from any specific strategy, treatment or therapy if a specific person tries such treatment or therapy mentioned in this book, or other media. The reader is advised to seek personalized advice from a qualified nutritionist, dietician, and/or other health care provider before attempting to implement information provided in this book.

Neither the author nor the publisher assumes any responsibility for any errors or omissions. The author and publisher also specifically disclaim any responsibility or liability resulting from the use of any of the information discussed in this book.

Other Books in the Inflammation Advisor Series

Eating Clean Recipes for Inflammation: Anti Inflammatory Diet Recipes

Best Gluten-Free Noodle Recipes: Rice and Quinoa Delights for the Gluten Challenged

Best Healthy Smoothie Recipes: Delicious Morning Smoothies to Start Your Day

Quick and Easy Low Fat Vegan Recipes: Simple Healthy Meals for the Hurried and Harried

Other Books by Dr. Iris Bell

Getting Whole, Getting Well: Healing Holistically from Chronic Illness

Chew on Things – It Helps You Think: Words of Wisdom from a Worried Canine

The Canine Art of Sleeping

Complete Self Help Program from "The Inflammation Advisor"

Fight Inflammatory Disease Naturally (4-module holistic program of natural solutions)

Visit http://ReducingInflammationNaturally.com

Table of Contents

Chapter 1 - What Is Inflammation?

Inflammation is the body's response to injury. You know that you are having inflammation when you experience redness, swelling, heat, and pain. It is the biochemical mediators and blood cells of the immune system in the body that cause these symptoms.

If you've ever sprained your ankle, you probably have felt it hurt, puff up like a balloon, get red and feel warm to the touch. That is how Nature tries to repair the damage in the short term.

For most people, short term (acute) inflammation is how you slow down, nourish and nurture the injured part, and recover. Acute inflammation usually contributes to a positive healing process.

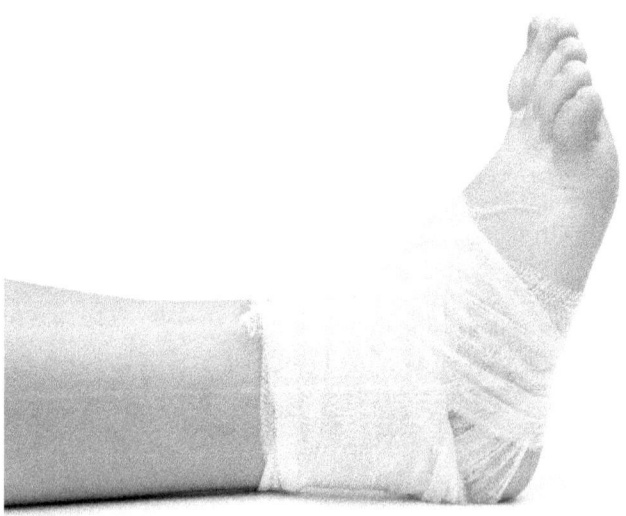

But, let's take a different situation. You develop daily severe abdominal pain with bloating and bloody diarrhea for months. Your doctor does some (not much fun) testing and concludes that you have a chronic condition called ulcerative colitis. This problem disrupts your life not for a few days, but every day. You may take prescription drugs, but these barely keep the lid on the discomfort and disruption you face all the time. You are not really cured – just controlled, sort of – in your symptoms.

Or, you develop daily severe joint pain and swelling. Over time, you notice that your joints in your hand are becoming distorted. The simple act of opening a jar, turning door knob, or dealing with multiple buttons on a shirt or blouse has become extremely painful and even impossible to accomplish. After an exam and multiple tests, your doctor tells you that you have an autoimmune disorder called rheumatoid arthritis.

These types of daily symptoms reflect chronic inflammation, that is, inflammation in the body that can lead to damage in organs and tissues over time. Somehow, things are triggering the mechanisms in the body that cause inflammation when the body really does not need to be inflamed. And the body cannot or does not stop the inflammation on its own.

Inflammation in Your Body

In fact, if your doctor has diagnosed you with a chronic health problem that ends in –itis, you probably have a condition that involves ongoing low grade inflammation. This can occur in many areas of the body. The precise symptoms you feel can differ from body part to part, but they all share an underlying inflammatory process.

The abnormalities that a doctor can find will depend on the

affected organs. Here is just a partial list of "–itis" inflammation-related health problems:

- Arthritis (joints)

- Dermatitis (skin)

- Cholangitis (gallbladder)

- Hepatitis (liver)

- Pancreatitis (pancreas)

- Gastritis (stomach)

- Esophagitis (esophagus)

- Colitis (intestines; colon)

- Bronchitis (lungs)

- Pericarditis (sac around the heart)

- Vasculitis (blood vessels)

- Myositis (muscles)

- Tendonitis (tendons)

- Thyroiditis (thyroid gland)

- Neuritis (nerves)

- Sinusitis (sinuses)

- Rhinitis (nose)

- Conjunctivitis, iritis, uveitis (eyes)

- Otitis (ears)

- Gingivitis (gums)

Your body is running its program for responding to injury – but in theory, there is no injury. Then the response itself creates damage over time. Usually the body has self regulatory mechanisms to counteract the effects of pro-inflammatory mediators as things heal.

But they are not producing healing on their own – and the inflammation just goes on and on, leading to tissue damage and a chronic inflammatory disease.

What causes chronic inflammation?

Why does this happen?

Sometimes you catch a virus and the immune system of the body is faked out into thinking that particular part of your body still has the virus in it – and so it attacks and attacks your own cells, trying to get rid of the "invader." Or the proteins in certain foods that you eat regularly trigger immune responses as if there were a dangerous material invading the body.

The "danger" is not "real" -- but your body interprets the information it receives from its environment as if the threat were very real. And, what happens instead of healing is that you end up with a chronic autoimmune disease.

Inflammation can be silent or can cause symptoms that grab your attention. A very general blood test for inflammation somewhere in the body is called the CRP (C-reactive protein) test. Doctors use it to monitor treatment progress in inflammatory conditions. Make sure you get your CRP level checked now, and ask for periodic re-checks to see if the treatments you are taking have helped.

Personalized Natural Treatment for Your Chronic Inflammation

Drugs are just going to cover over the problems, that is, suppress them, trying to hold the "invader" or "threat" in check. The disease-altering drugs for rheumatoid arthritis, for instance, can knock down your inflammatory mediators to lessen symptoms.

However, the price you pay for that treatment approach is distorting the normal ability of your body to respond to infections that invade or cancer cells that develop in your body. That is a serious price to pay – trading one bad problem for another.

The drugs are not intended to address what sets off the body's inflammatory processes in the first place. Sadly, most conventional doctors are not trained and don't have time to look for those hidden types of causes. It takes a different set of questions and some detective work to sort the deeper causes out and undo the damage.

So, the answer to what causes chronic inflammatory symptoms is going to be found beyond the mechanisms of the inflammation itself. We have to look at the environment. The whole environment of the individual person. You and your interactions with your world.

What is your environment anyway? It includes psychological, social, physical, chemical, and biological factors. Yes, that includes stress from your work, family, and personal life. It includes how nurturing or non-nurturing your environment was for you in your early years. But, your environment and your stressors are a lot more than psychosocial. Stress as people usually think about it is just the tip of the iceberg.

What exactly do you eat? What exactly do you breathe? What do you put in and on your body every day? What chemicals, dusts, molds, and pollens do you encounter in your everyday life in your personal clothing, hygiene, home and work settings? Foods, chemicals, dusts, molds and pollens – as well as drugs -- are also environmental stressors.

If you live in a developed country, you probably spend 90% of your day indoors. What is in the air you breathe and the water you drink and bathe in? Have you managed to pick up some chronic infections like Lyme disease (from ticks) or parasites or pathological fungi or yeasts?

Maybe you are "lucky" and the various symptoms that make you miserable all the time don't have a disease label – yet. That's good news – you can take action before you get a label. You do not want an –itis label. When you get one, you are probably already suffering a lot of damage from inflammation. Your silent inflammation has gotten very noisy and loud, so to speak.

You are embedded in your environment. That is the nature of Nature. To the extent you control your environment, you can go a long way toward controlling your health and well-being. I am not talking about global warming here (that's a bigger and different debate).

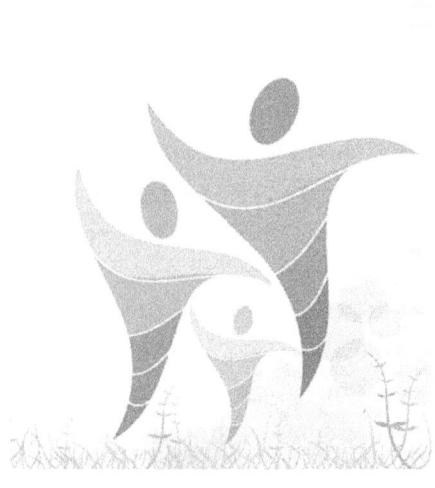

I am talking about your little personal environment. Inside and outside your body. The one that matters the most to you day to day. The one that you can control.

If you don't look into these questions at it all, figure out the biggest factors in your inner and outer environments that trigger your chronic inflammation, and do something about them, you may end up with a chronic downhill course of pain, disability, and even, in some cases, death.

Summary and Conclusions

The basic principles you will find are:

- Remove the triggers

- Replenish the nutrients

- Restore the balance in the biochemistry of the body and the overall system

There is no simple cause or easy fix, no matter what some people claim. But there are good solutions. Even great solutions. They require you take an active part in your own recovery. Healing from a chronic illness is not a spectator sport. Even if you feel pretty tired and worn out and hardly ready to get in the game.

To recover, to heal – you must get in the game. Play as if your life depends on it.

Because it does.

In coming chapters, we will talk about the best foods and worst foods to eat, addictive foods and why they can cancel benefits from an otherwise "healthy" food for your particular body, natural anti inflammatory supplements (vitamins, minerals, herbs), mind-body techniques, and other holistic approaches.

The rest of this book and our complete "Fight Inflammatory Disease Naturally" Program (www.ReducingInflammationNaturally.com) are all about solutions.

As Mother Teresa said, "Let us begin."

"Yesterday is gone. Tomorrow has not yet come. We have only today. Let us begin."

-- Mother Teresa

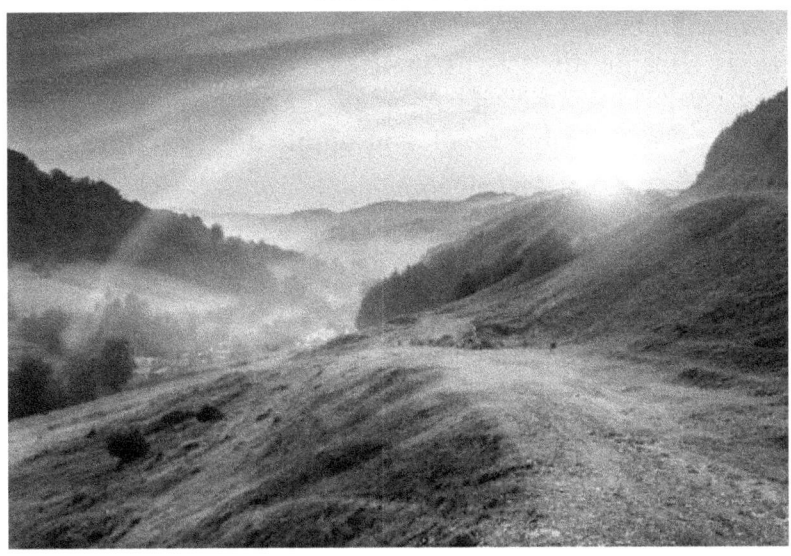

Chapter 2 – Anti Inflammatory Diet

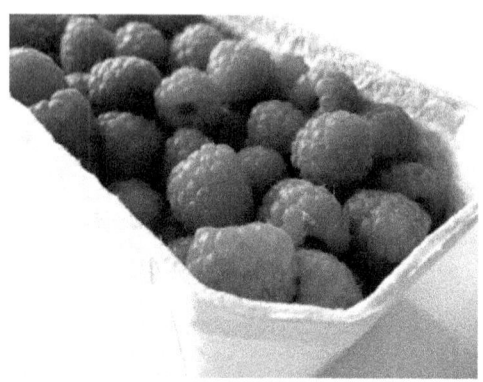

There is no single anti-inflammatory diet, but most versions of an anti-inflammatory diet have certain components in common. Sometimes you may hear it called the wellness diet or Mediterranean Diet. This diet does not have a flashy name yet, unlike so many trendy diets that come and go.

This is really a long-term lifestyle eating plan. The basic philosophy behind the anti-inflammatory diet is very simple.

There are certain foods that are known to cause inflammation flare-ups, and then there are other foods that actually help the body reduce inflammation. This is important because inflammation has been linked to some serious chronic diseases that produce health problems and even sometimes, death. A good anti-inflammatory diet includes the desirable foods and eliminates the undesirable foods.

Understanding Inflammation

Inflammation is a biological process in which the body's white blood cells and certain biochemicals react to injury and illness to help protect and heal our bodies. However, in certain situations, such as arthritis, the body triggers an inflammatory response that attempts to fight off foreign substances that are not present. There are certain foods that contribute to inflammatory response. The anti-inflammatory diet is designed around reducing foods that promote inflammation in many people while eating food that helps reduce it.

Reducing Inflammation through Proper Nutrition

Inflammation has been linked to a number of chronic conditions, such as depression, heart disease, diabetes, arthritis, and cancer. This makes the ability to effectively control inflammation extremely important. Proper nutrition plays a major role in holistic health, which includes blood glucose levels, cholesterol levels, hormonal imbalances and more. Proper nutrition also has the potential to help lower high inflammation levels.

There are two primary ways to approach an anti-inflammatory diet — (a) the avoidance or elimination and (b) the specific food addition approach. The elimination phase refers to identifying and avoiding certain foods that promote inflammatory responses in your body. The food addition approach is to find foods that actually help to reduce inflammation, and then incorporate them into your diet.

Foods to Avoid

The key is to identify certain foods in your diet that may be contributing to your inflammation issues. Below are some of the most common foods that are known to cause inflammation.

- The three Ps — packaged, processed and prepared foods. Fast food types usually fall into this category. The high level of sugars, flavor enhancers like MSG (monosodium glutamate, now often hidden by manufacturers' food labels with other names such as hydrolyzed vegetable protein or hydrolyzed yeast), food additives, preservatives, and artificial sweeteners in fast food make them foods that are highly toxic — capable of triggering inflammatory responses.

- Hydrogenated and trans fats — found in foods such as shortening, lard, margarine or any products or foods made with them. This includes many baked goods such as cookies, cakes and pies. There are healthier alternatives for making all these foods.

- Red meats, especially animal proteins such as processed red meats, will produce some level of inflammation. Some experts suggest that meat should be treated as a secondary food instead of the main dish. Processed meats are especially risky for long term health problems. There are healthier forms of animal proteins such as wild caught fish that are preferable for many individuals.

- Fried foods — are not only highly inflammatory, but they may contribute to a number of other health issues, such as coronary heart disease, high cholesterol and more.

- White sugar — is another culprit that not only exacerbates inflammation conditions in the body but can create blood sugar spikes and aftereffects that lead to insulin resistance.

- Other foods to which people with chronic inflammation are often sensitive include corn, egg, wheat/rye/barley, yeast, and milk/dairy products, nightshade vegetables such as tomatoes and potatoes.

- These foods might be produced in a healthy organic way, but the natural constituents of the specific food can still trigger inflammatory responses in susceptible individuals.

These are examples of the foods that you should avoid.

Foods that Help Reduce Inflammation

Just as the foods mentioned above can cause inflammation flares, the following foods usually have the capacity to lower the level of inflammation in the body.

- **Good oils**: The number of these good oils is growing. Obviously, you want to have oils such as fish oil, krill oil and unfiltered olive oil, but there are other oils that were once believed to be unhealthy but now research suggests that they are actually good for you.

  - One example is coconut oil. It has a number of benefits, one of which is the reduction of inflammation.

- **Fish**: It is important to distinguish the difference between farm raised fish and wild caught fish, such as snapper, salmon, cod, tuna,* halibut and bass. Buy it fresh and ask the market to clarify if it is wild caught.

  - The omega-3 fatty acids found in these fish

are loaded with antioxidants that will help to reduce inflammation.

- o Tuna has an asterisk (*) next to it because of the increased levels of the heavy metal mercury that this fish can contain. Some experts claim that light tuna is somewhat less mercury contaminated compared with white tuna, but overall this means that you should limit how much of this specific type of fish you eat.

- **Nuts and fruits**: Nuts and fresh fruits make a good in between meal snack. Nuts, such as almonds, hazelnuts, walnuts, pistachios and sunflower seeds are great choices to help lower your body's inflammation level.

  - o Peanuts are actually a legume and are not necessarily a good "nut" for these purposes. Many people are severely allergic to peanuts.

  - o Again, with any food, even if it is healthy for people in general, you as an individual may be sensitive to it and need to avoid it.

A wealth of information continues to surface through numerous studies that reveal the value of anti-inflammatory diets such as the Mediterranean Diet. A study conducted by the Harvard School of Public Health revealed that the Mediterranean Diet helped reduce the risk of heart disease among young American workers. Even when these people were sedentary and did not exercise, the benefits were still detectable.

Inflammation is a major health concern, and one of the most powerful tools that you have against it is your diet. What you choose to take into your body as well as what you refuse to allow into your body will play a major role in your ability to control your inflammation levels.

Your Action Steps

- Keep a 3-day food diet of everything you eat and drink – meals, snacks, beverages.

- Go back through this diet diary and write down the ingredients of any packaged or processed foods. If you eat farm caught fish, ask what coloring or other chemicals might be added to improve its appearance and taste.

- Replace any processed and packaged foods with unprocessed, raw or lightly cooked forms of the food, as appropriate to the type of food. Go for simple in the first stages, not elaborate recipes. You still do not really know what foods might trigger inflammation in you as an individual. That step comes next.

Chapter 3 – Hidden Food Addictions and Their Pro-Inflammatory Effects

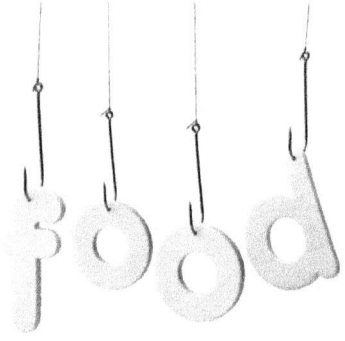

The flip side of food allergies/sensitivities/intolerance is sometimes food addiction. This is the compulsive eating of foods. The addiction actually creates cycles of ups and downs in your mood and physical symptoms.

Intense food cravings and, often, binges can be part of the larger problem. Food binging can be as secretive as any alcoholic's or drug addict's binges. In fact, one clue to foods that trigger your addictive eating may be in the foods from which your favorite alcoholic beverages are made – barley, wheat, corn, yeast, grapes, or potato, for instance.

You often do not realize that you are a food addict. This can also involve foods that you eat every day, as part of your regular diet. Certainly, obvious types of foods like sweets containing table sugar or sucrose or dextrose (corn sugar) are especially addictive.

The foods to suspect first are ones that make the reward centers of your brain happy and are quickly absorbed into your system to give you a literal rush or pick-me-up. You could be addicted to a long list of frequently-eaten foods and not know it.

Eating these foods may temporarily make you feel better. You might even get a short pick-me-up from eating a snack food that contains foods you are addicted to. Chocolate chip cookies, for instance, could include wheat, cane sugar, beet sugar, or corn sugar, chocolate, egg, and milk. Lots of goodies for your reward pathways in the brain – but the foods themselves then set off inflammatory reactions in the body.

If eating a food *seems* to relieve your afternoon fatigue or dullness or even makes a daily headache go away for a while, you may have found a trigger food. The ability of any food to change symptoms that you experience often is a warning sign of hidden food addiction. Instead of relying on the food to keep you on a cycle of eating for symptom relief and then going into withdrawal symptoms – and eating the food again and again for temporary improvement, stop eating it all together.

If you feel cravings coming on, you have found a food (and its possibly multiple ingredients), that could be causing your chronic symptoms. Do a simple test – eliminate all forms of that food for 4 or 5 to 7 days. Consider yourself just like a heroin addict, because that food may be playing on the same brain chemicals and receptors that are involved in drug addiction. Literally like drug addiction.

If you get through 5-7 days completely off the specific food, you can experience firsthand that this situation is going on for you. After this brief avoidance period, you can do a test -- eat a single meal of all you want of the single specific recently-avoided food. Record symptoms for the next 24 hours.

An offending food on a challenge test will set off a more noticeable short term worsening of your chronic symptoms. You will have unmasked a hidden food addiction.

The trouble is, every time you eat a source of the food(s) you are addicted to, you feed the addiction. You keep a cycle going. When the effects of the snack wear off, you develop withdrawal symptoms. You might feel sluggish and tired. You can't think straight. Maybe you get headaches. Until the next snack.

Then the whole cycle starts all over again.

You may not be an alcoholic or a drug addict – but you could be a food addict. To different extents, we all have our brains wired for adaptive changes that can bring about addictive behaviors.

What Foods Can Be Addictive?

Some of the commonly-eaten foods that can be offending or trigger foods for you are corn and corn sugar, wheat, yeast, milk, egg, beef, white potato, cane sugar, beet sugar, and chocolate. For you, the list may go on from there. Some children may have only a few trigger foods, but adults with chronic illnesses often have multiple offenders in their diets to identify and avoid.

Many "junk foods" are addictive, but so are healthier versions of a particular food for a specific individual. For instance, the best organic whole wheat product can still be addictive, if the person is sensitized to wheat in any form.

Foods like wheat naturally include proteins like gluten that the gut breaks down into opiate-like chemicals called exorphins (you may have heard of endorphins, the opiate-like brain transmitters that can produce a runner's high). Exorphins are named as they are in that their source is from outside the body (exo-) but their effects are like those of heroin or morphine. It is more complex than opiate-like effects as well.

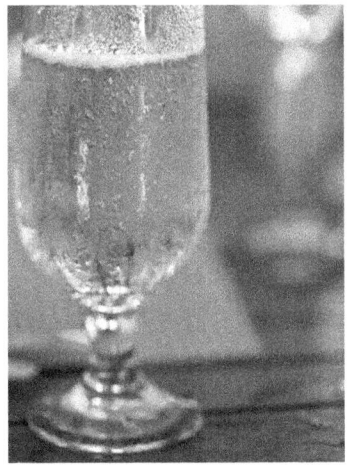

Addiction involves multiple interactive pathways in the brain, external cues to give in to addictive behaviors, and social factors from the people you spend time around. Far more things contribute to food addictions, like other types of addictions, than just the food or drug, the brain, or the immune system per se.

In terms of foods, it doesn't stop there. There are people who get addicted to all sorts of other foods, including some fruits or vegetables, various other types of animal proteins, beans, or soy.

The faster absorbed the food, the more likely it is to set this addictive cycle into motion. Believe it or not, some people may prefer beer because of the interaction of the alcohol with the food sources from which it is made, such as barley (which is a close relative to wheat), brewers yeast, and hops.

Someone else may enjoy wine because of the interaction of the alcohol (which is absorbed super fast) with the food source like grapes (and sugar in grapes) and other fermented foods (like yeast).

You may have heard about "sugar addiction" or "chronic systemic "yeast" infections. Often, the problems are more complex for people who have those types of health issues.

They probably have many additional food addictions/sensitivities/intolerances (the flip side of a food addiction is a food sensitivity or intolerance) that they don't even recognize.

These may not be classical "allergies" in terms of their mechanisms (they don't use an antibody called IgE to occur), but their effects can be just as devastating and worse for your health and quality of life. Most allergists do not consider this type of health problem within their scope of practice. Instead, you can find help from naturopathic doctors and some integrative MDs as well (see the Resources list at the end of this book).

Testing for Addictive Trigger Foods

Testing for trigger foods is the best (and cheapest) way to figure out if you have a food addiction problem. A trigger food test requires you to eliminate all sources of the item from your diet for 5-7 days. Then eat a test meal of only that single food (no extra condiments or other foods in the meal). The only beverage with a food test meal is plain water.

Keep a food trigger journal of what you eat, when you eat it, and what happens in the 1-24 hours after the test meal. If the test item is a trigger food, you will likely have unmasked your addiction and will experience the food intolerance side of the story.

In other words, the test meal will cause a set of symptoms you had commonly experienced in the past. You mood might flip around from irritability to depression for no apparent reason. A few hours later, you might get fatigued and headachy. Your heart may feel like it is racing. After that, you

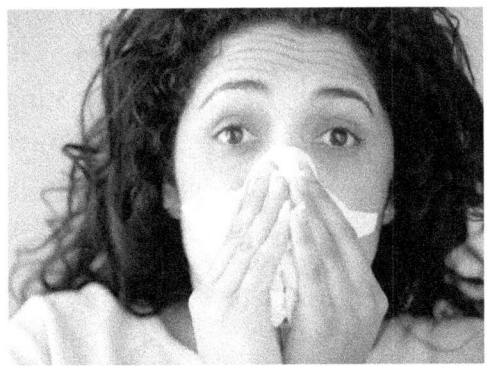

might find your nose running for a while.

By the next day, all of that amazing sequence of symptoms could be gone, if you do not eat another meal containing the trigger food. This is not a simple switch to turn symptoms on and off, but on average, you can begin to sort out which foods are major triggers and which ones are safe or safer for you to eat.

Also remember that during pollen season, you may find that you temporarily do not tolerate certain foods that are marginal or OK the rest of the year. Just avoid them for the duration of the pollen season and go back to careful use in your diet the rest of the time.

Some foods are a little slow or delayed in triggering you – so you might need to do two consecutive test meals of something like wheat cereal (you can make this from hot wheat cereal with nothing added).

Overall, trigger food tests can give you awareness that how previously unsuspected foods have been playing a role in chronic health problems of all types.

What's in it for you? Eliminating trigger foods will help you feel energetic, alert, clear-headed, and less likely to experience chronic physical symptoms like indigestion, headaches, fatigue, depression, muscle and joint pains.

An added benefit of figuring our your individual trigger foods is that eliminating them may help you stick to your weight loss diet and even lose weight that you can keep off. Otherwise when people go on diets and then return to eating their addictive foods right after they reach their target weight, they reactivate the addictive cycle and regain the weight.

Big note of caution: If you happen to have serious medical conditions such as (but not limited to) asthma or epilepsy, do not attempt food tests without close medical supervision. You simply may not be able to try direct food ingestion tests.

It is very possible that a trigger food for you could set off a bad asthma attack or epileptic seizure. So, as every reader should, you especially need to discuss your options with your doctor before trying to test any foods.

An alternative option for people in whom food testing by eating (ingestion tests) are too dangerous is to ask your doctor or naturopath to run some specialized blood tests such as a mediator release test, IgG food allergy test, and IgE food allergy test.

The results can be useful as a starting place to eliminate likely major offenders, but usually not quite as accurate as the ingestion testing. Still, these can put you on the right track toward feeling better from less inflammation in the body.

Using the Results of Your Trigger Food Tests

Once you identify a food that can set off symptoms, put it on the list to eliminate from your diet completely for at least 3 months. You can re-test it after the 3 month avoidance period ends. The intensity of the reactivity after avoidance begins can start to diminish as early as 3 weeks afterwards.

After several months of avoidance, you may be able to resume eating some of your trigger foods in a very limited way. That is, you may be able to get by when you are limiting the frequency of use, that is, no more often than once in 4 or 5 to 7 days. By limiting frequency of use, sometimes you can avoid reactivating the addictive cycle and the chronic inflammatory symptoms that go along with it.

Learn to think in terms of timing, not just amounts of food. Addiction is set into motion by repeated intermittent use, which also masks its development and leaves the affected person in an endless cycle of ups and downs in mood and health.

If you again experience a flare of symptoms after a food re-test, leave it out of your diet again for another 3 months.

Keep re-checking how you stand with the food every few months until it appears OK to put back into your diet *occasionally*. "Occasionally" means just that – no more often than once in 4 or 5 to 7 days.

The most important point about reintroducing a food to which you were addicted and/or intolerant is to make sure that you do not slip back into eating the food every day. Frequency of use makes a difference.

If you resume eating a trigger food daily, you'll slip back into the addictive cycle – craving the food, feeling better temporarily when you eat it, and then getting withdrawal symptoms when its effects wear off. The cycle will come on gradually – you might not even realize what is happening until you step back and acknowledge that you are addicted...again. The symptoms return, and the weight piles on...again.

It's actually like a heroin or opiate addict in endless cycles of highs and withdrawals. After a while, the highs are harder to get from a hit of the drugs, and it takes more of the drug to get high.

As a food addict, you eventually run into the same inability to get the "pick-me-ups" that the food used to bring. Eventually, you spend most of your time with the food intolerance/withdrawal side of the problem – the unpleasant physical symptoms, fatigue, and negative moods.

Food addiction is not just a metaphor. It is a real biological effect. Scientists have already shown that they can get animals addicted to table sugar (sucrose) – and it cross-sensitizes the same brain chemistry that amphetamine or cocaine can affect. The sugar-addicted animals get withdrawal symptoms and crave sugar just as much as a drug addict craves their drug of choice.

Sugar is not the only food with direct links to the brain chemistry of addiction. You may have heard about runners' highs. Intense exercise can activate endorphins and make an athlete feel exhilarated from running. Some runners will even admit to feeling addicted to exercise, experiencing withdrawal symptoms when an injury or bad weather prevents them from getting their daily "hit" from exercise.

Just as a runner might get into an addictive cycle to activate their internal endorphins, a food addict might end up caught in their own addictive cycle -- caused by the exorphins from the digestion of not only gluten-containing wheat and related grains, but also from casein proteins in milk.

Then you also have to contend with the release of internal brain endorphins that eating sweet or fatty foods can naturally trigger. Since the gut contains enzymes that digest proteins like gluten in wheat, rye, and barley or casein in milk into exorphins, you do not need to be gluten-sensitive in an immune sense to have trouble from gluten- or dairy-containing foods.

What Food Addiction Means for You on a Diet

Although it is true that some people have genetic tendencies to be overweight, your genes are NOT your destiny. Unless you let them be. New research shows that environmental and diet factors turn genes on and off. In short, what you eat plays with your genes, turning sets of them on and off. The whole field of epigenetics in medical research is now focused on how to use epigenetic adaptive changes to our advantage for healing from disease.

Choosing the right non-addictive foods for you is likely to tilt the balance in your favor – to flip the switches on your genes in a good way for health and normal weight. This could be the missing step toward setting yourself up for reducing inflammation and perhaps successful weight loss for the first time.

So, what does this all mean for you as someone wanting to diet successfully? It means at least two main things:

1. You cannot hope to lose as much weight as you might otherwise if you keep addictive trigger foods and beverages in your diet. These foods can lead to

inflammation, pain, and water weight gain.

2. The tough time that you have in the first few days to a week of any new diet is not just from reducing calories – it's literally from food withdrawal. Your brain chemistry is making you crave the eliminated foods.

The initial dieting blues/misery could be severe withdrawal symptoms from your trigger foods. The good news is that if you go into the diet armed with knowledge about which foods you absolutely must avoid, you can make the transition to a healthier diet a lot easier.

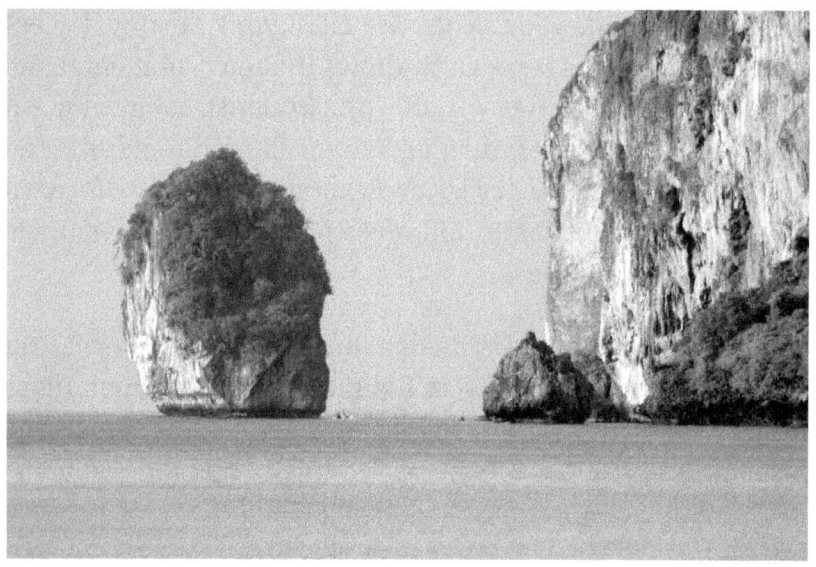

You need to realize that you are between a rock and a hard place – sure, your cravings for the addictive food are powerful, but your chronic inflammatory symptoms are miserable. What are you willing to do to get through a temporary period of suffering to relieve a lifetime of deteriorating health from inflammation?

In fact, you probably would want to identify your main trigger foods with food testing before you try adding anti-inflammatory supplements or going on a weight loss diet of any form.

While many natural supplements are invaluable in combating inflammation, they are usually made from herbs or foods. They themselves, while chemically good for you in theory, might trigger adverse effects until your system settles down over a period of months of a simpler eating style.

Trying to rely just on anti-inflammatory natural supplements or drugs while still eating major food triggers for your chronic inflammation is like trying to put on perfume to cover up the fact that you haven't bathed in a week. It's just never enough to fix the issue completely.

Once you have found the problem foods and eliminated them (or replaced them with non-addictive alternatives – e.g., plain brown rice-based rice cakes if you have problems from wheat and yeast based breads), your overall anti inflammatory program is going to go much more smoothly.

From taking action on this food addiction factor alone, you can make a big dent in the pro-inflammatory factors that keep you stuck in your personal situation.

What If This Gets Too Hard to Do On Your Own?

Can't take the withdrawal symptoms from foods? While natural supplements may not always be a first choice, other holistic strategies can be a big help.

Find yourself a good local acupuncturist for supporting your system through the changes in diet. Acupuncture is not a cover up – it is a rebalancing of your whole system. It can help reduce your tendency toward addictive eating and toward the experience of your chronic inflammatory symptoms.

One place to begin looking for a good acupuncturist is at www.AcuFinder.com. Acupuncture can help with many different types of addictions and related symptoms. Some studies show that acupuncture can even help alcoholics and drug addicts get through their withdrawal periods more easily.

Remember – it is also often the case that complete elimination of a specific food for a period of 3-6 months or so can lower your sensitization level and allow you to reintroduce the food on a limited basis in terms of frequency without setting off the cravings.

Just do not try to go back to eating "just a little" every day or two – "too often" is worse than "too much" in the food addiction world.

As we emphasized above, if you do the elimination period and a test meal 3 months later still sets off cravings and symptom cycling, eliminate the food for another few months before re-testing.

Your Action Steps:

1. Talk to your doctor or primary health care provider about whether or not it would be safe for you to try some trigger food tests at home.

2. Eliminate each food that you discover to be a trigger food for mood swings, physical symptoms, fatigue, or pain (joint pain, muscle pain).

Leave it out of your diet plan for 3 months before you re-test it. Keep a detailed trigger food and symptom diary.

3. Replace a problem food with a rarely-eaten item that you have not been eating very often.

So, for instance, you might find that rice based pastas, breads, etc. are OK, even if wheat based foods are not. Try almond milk instead of cow's milk if milk is an issue for you.

Is beef a factor in your joint pain? Rotate in some wild game meats like venison or elk, fish and turkey instead.

4. Consider getting a specialized food sensitivity/intolerance blood test for multiple foods and food additives.

If you cannot figure out all of the possible triggers or it is simply not safe for you to test foods by elimination and challenge eating tests, ask your doctor or naturopath for a specialized blood test for all types of adverse food reactions, not just IgE types of reactions. Visit our sister website at http://foodaddictionsecrets.com for more resources.

5. Get even more in-depth help with food addiction.

Visit http://OvercomeFoodAddiction.com for other resources, news, updates, and a complete membership program.

Some people with food addictions need to go onto a complete rotation diet in which no food or food in the same biological food family is eaten more often than once in 4 or 5 to 7 days. Meals start off simple to keep the body from initiating or triggering intolerance or addictive responses.

Chapter 4 – Your Personal Environment – Pro- or Anti Inflammatory?

Hidden sensitivities and intolerances that can trigger chronic inflammation in the body do not stop with foods. Have you been getting headaches, sinus pressure, runny nose, experiencing fatigue, dizzy spells, digestive issues, joint or muscle pain, palpitations in your chest and/or difficulties breathing?

Have you gone to doctors hoping that they will figure out what is wrong with you but still do not have any answers? Is your new diet program helping, but not quite enough to clear everything up?

People may be telling you that your symptoms are all in your head or that you simply "just" have allergies. You may be frustrated because you are certain there is something more wrong with you, but expensive and extensive tests have not turned up answers you can use. If this all sounds painfully familiar, you may also have some form of multiple chemical sensitivity syndrome or MCS. Some types of MCS-like conditions are called environmentally-related illnesses.

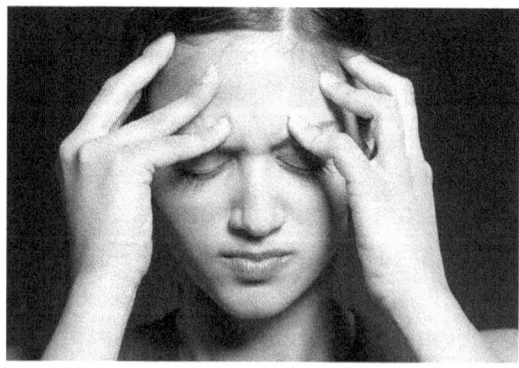

One of the reasons some physicians may not be so quick to make the diagnosis of MCS is because there is still much controversy surrounding what some call "environmental illness." Doctors have little to no training in clinical issues in environmentally-related illnesses.

Many experts, including the American Medical Association have said "the connection(s) between the patient's symptoms and environmental exposures are speculative and evidence of disease is lacking."

Many physicians simply chalk these symptoms up as allergies or even hypochondriasis. That does not help anyone suffering unexplained symptoms. Sometimes patients get referrals to psychiatrists or psychologists, who can help a person cope better, but not usually to sort out the medical aspects of their problems.

Psychiatrists themselves often realize that environmentally-ill patients seem to have clinical problems that go beyond what treating stress, anxiety or depression can help. Patient surveys indicate that chemically-sensitive individuals often report that antidepressant and antianxiety drugs made them sicker.

This is not to reject every type of psychiatric/psychological care – see the chapter on valuable mind-body therapies for useful options. Improving any chronically ill person's sense of empowerment and control can promote healing and recovery.

The actual scientific evidence supports some common sense ideas – that is, even if a person is anxious or depressed, environmental exposure may still be setting off additional symptoms or contributing directly to change in brain chemistry involved in anxiety and depression. This is an important avenue for possible treatment and it deserves serious consideration.

If you, however, are one who suffers, you know that MCS is a "real" illness that can be quite debilitating. Besides the above symptoms listed above, you may also be experiencing congestion, headaches, chest pain, palpitations, rashes, muscle and joint soreness, sleeping problems and even memory trouble and inability to concentrate.

While some experts believe that there are no methods of properly diagnosing or treating MCS and other environmentally-related illnesses, there are still things that can be done in order to determine if you are having some sort of reaction to certain chemicals in your environment.

Types of Testing

As with food triggers, a first step in trying to determine if you have chemical intolerances (if present, there are usually more than one) or MCS is to make a list of all of the pollutants or chemicals that you have been exposed to or to which chemicals you are currently being exposed.

Some of these chemicals include: pesticides and herbicides, cigarette smoke, perfumes, paints, carpets and carpet pads, wood burning stoves, sulfur dioxide and other air pollutants such as exhaust from automobiles. Besides these air pollutants, there are also chemicals found in household supplies such as soaps and detergents and even in the foods that you eat, especially fruits and vegetables that have been sprayed with pesticides and grown with chemical fertilizers.

Some tests can help you to determine what kinds of chemicals to which your body is more sensitive. These include selective skin tests, routine lab tests including a nasal smear, chemical toxicity screening tests, mediator release testing, lung function measurements and a neurologic examination. Look into even more specialized testing that ordinary clinical laboratories and doctors may not consider (see Resources List at the end of this book and on our website at http://InflammationAdvisor.com/resources) for details).

Make sure to ask for a red blood cell magnesium level test. Many people with chemical sensitivities seem to run chronically low in magnesium levels. This vital mineral plays a key role in reducing anxiety, improving sleep quality, and preventing muscle spasms and cramps as well as lessening the risk of certain types of palpitations.

Other, often controversial tests that can be done include specialized blood tests for environmental chemical triggers, provocation testing using sublingual drops or antigen injections just under the skin, muscle resistance testing and avoidance programs where you simply avoid certain chemicals for a period of time. More in depth environmental quality testing can also be done in the home and in the workplace to determine which chemicals are present.

Finding out which chemicals you are sensitive to is a huge first step in getting well. There is no magic pill that doctors can prescribe to cure MCS or to simply mask its symptoms; however, there are things you can do to rid yourself completely of some or all of the symptoms you may be experiencing.

For instance if you have identified that ammonia in the cleaning supplies that you use to clean your home is triggering a symptom, then you know to simply avoid using that product. As chemical sensitivities are becoming more and more common, there are many products that are more clean or natural without any added fumes or dyes.

While these products may not always be found at your local retail outlet, they can be found online or at a store that specializes in organic materials. Some other products you may need to avoid include scented products such as perfume or cologne, air fresheners, paint, scented fabric softeners, chlorine, new carpeting, and personal care products like hairspray and soap.

If you have a new smelly carpet in your home or office, at least speed up the outgassing by opening the doors and windows and airing out the space. If you have no way to air it out, consider trying a carpet odor absorbant that captures the volatile organic compounds that new carpet releases (http://www.cleartheair.com/english/new_carpet_odors.ht ml).

Avoiding Trigger Chemicals and Finding Safer Alternatives

Stop having pesticide services or garden herbicide treatments in and around your home. These agents are linked with serious health problems from Parkinson's disease to cancers to childhood developmental conditions.

You can find alternative approaches that you will personally need to test to see if you tolerate them. Our Resources page (http://InflammationAdvisor.com/resources) lists a number of possibilities, and it is updated periodically.

If you have natural gas heating and/or a gas stove, look seriously at switching over to an all-electric house. Costs are not necessarily much higher to do so. Even with modern switches and controls, even low levels of natural gas in the home air breathing environment can trigger symptoms in people with a high degree of sensitivity to chemicals.

Use products that do not contain additives like fragrances, alcohol, nitrates, plastic compounds, phenol and formaldehyde. Beware that many common household items such as make-up , facial tissue, toilet paper, feminine hygiene products, enamels, and even fabrics such as bedding and clothes contain chemicals such as formaldehyde.

While avoiding the above products, you will be helping yourself immensely but there is still more than you can do to alleviate symptoms of MCS. It can be helpful to make sure your home is properly vented and it is a good idea to open up the windows for at least ten minutes a day.

In the kitchen, decide to use electric appliances like an electric stove as opposed to a gas stove. Add a good drinking water filter for cooking, drinking, and showering. You do not want to volatilize chlorine during hot showers, for instance, but you can avoid that issue by adding a good water filter onto your shower.

Even de-cluttering your home helps. Try to clear out newspapers and other printed materials, empty boxes and unused items.

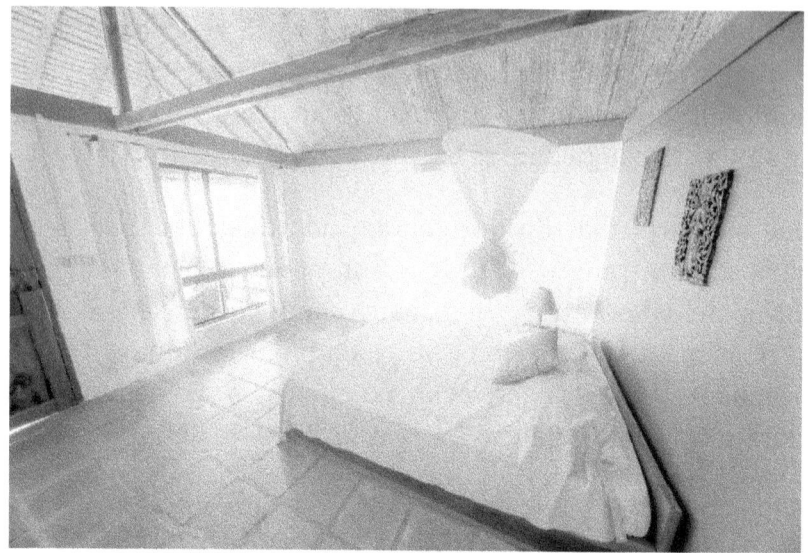

Make sure that you set up a "clean and safe" room such as your bedroom, where you spend at least 8 hours each day. There your bed and bedding should be organic cotton, wool, silk or other natural, undyed products that you tolerate. Choose metal, glass, or real wood furniture whenever possible.

The flooring should be tile. Try for metal or natural wood furniture, not pressboard, which outgasses formaldehyde and other volatile organic chemicals that contribute to chronic illnesses. Laminate flooring may still outgas some chemicals. Properly sealed real wood floors should be OK.

Avoid wall-to-wall carpeting and even flooring laminates for their chemical outgassing. Avoid piling up books and papers in the room. Cotton throw rugs are OK. Air outdoors and then keep dry-cleaned clothes elsewhere in the house, not your bedroom closet.

You may want to swap out bedrooms for a simpler bedroom

in the house to avoid having an en suite bathroom that could expose you to mold and mold toxins from water leaks from sinks, showers, bathtubs, or toilets.

Get a high quality air filter/purifier for at least your bedroom, where you will spend at least 8 hours per day. Higher end brands that do a very good job with chemicals in indoor air include: IQ Air, Austin Air, and Alen Air Purifiers.

The practical reality is not that you can completely avoid environmental chemicals. Rather, this approach stems from the idea that we each have a personal total load of exposures from foods, chemicals, pollens, dusts, molds, and medications. What are the biggest sources of exposures that trigger your symptoms?

Start with eliminating or at least reducing those sources, then move on to others. You may be pleasantly surprised to find that you tolerate less avoidable exposures if you stay away from your own personal big triggers.

Basic principle – air out new items that put out chemical odors, leaving them outdoors or in a less-used space until the smell is gone. For items that can be laundered, wash them repeatedly until the odor leaves the fabric before wearing or using them in your personal space. Borax is a good mold retardant, and there are other helpful products as well.

There is hope for those who suffer with environmentally-related illnesses or MCS. If you take the time and energy to pinpoint which chemicals are individual triggers for your symptoms, you will feel much better and may even find yourself recovering enough to enjoy a much happier quality of life.

Your Action Steps:

1. **Take stock of your home, work, and/or school environments, indoors and outdoors**. Be complete and comprehensive in your list of possible exposures.

2. **Identify specific concrete changes that you can make** in your bedroom and home to clear out sources of chemicals, dusts, and molds. Consider ways in which you may be able to modify your work or school environments to reduce chemical exposures.

3. **Purchase a good indoor air purifier** to clean the air in your immediate breathing space. Make sure that it includes at least a HEPA filter to capture the most important environmental triggers for your inflammatory response.

Chapter 5 – Natural Anti Inflammatory Supplements

Natural anti-inflammatory supplements are a core part of the overall program for reducing inflammation naturally.

As you may know, many of the pharmaceutical drugs used to treat inflammation have negative side effects. Ibuprofen and other NSAIDs (nonsteroidal anti-inflammatory drugs) can cause irritation and even bleeding of the stomach as well as damage to the kidneys. Additionally, these drugs block the mechanisms of inflammation that cause symptoms, but they do not treat the underlying causes of inflammation.

This is why the food addiction/sensitivity and personal environment methods to eliminate exposures to your own triggers are so important. Before you try to suppress the inflammatory process, try to avoid setting it off in the first place.

In addition, at the root of many chronic inflammatory disorders is an imbalance and/or insufficiency in nutritional intake for your individual situation. Natural supplements are therefore a safer and more effective treatment for inflammation.

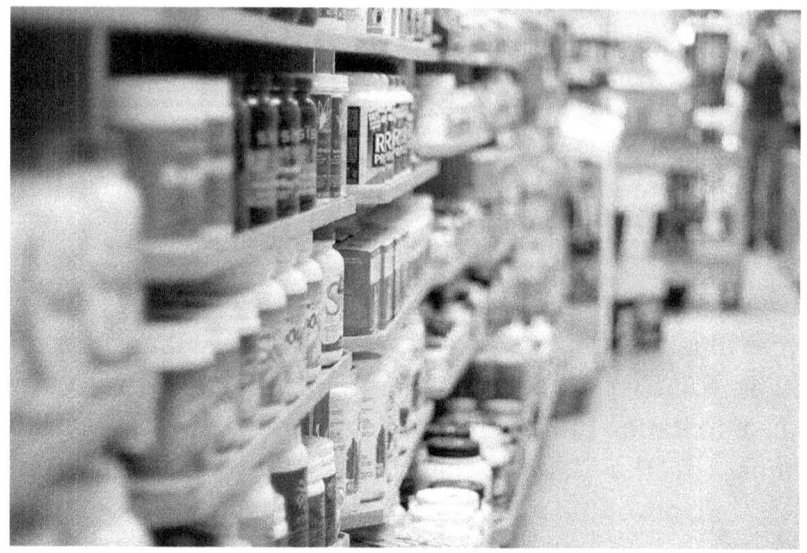

Natural Anti Inflammatory Supplement Options

Omega-3 fatty acids are important in any diet, and they especially help with inflammatory disorders. An excess of omega-6 fatty acids is one of the primary causes of inflammation, and these fatty acids are common in processed foods. However, ingesting more omega-3 can neutralize the negative effects of omega-6.

Omega-3 reduces the risk of cancer and asthma by lowering inflammation in the body. You can get your daily dose of omega-3 from fish oil capsules, which are available in most vitamin aisles.

Vitamin D3 is a hormone-like vitamin that our skin can make if exposed to sunlight long enough daily. But, with the indoor lives of most modern people and the widespread use of sunscreens to protect against skin cancer, a huge proportion of the population is dangerously low or deficient in vitamin D. Among the many health risks of low vitamin D levels are inflammatory skin conditions, asthma, arthritis, diabetes, and cancer.

Current recommendations may not be enough to get your blood level into an optimal range for the anti-inflammatory effects of this essential nutrient. Rather than just 800 IU/day, many people may need doses closer to 5,000 IU/day or more to achieve levels around 50-60 ng/ml. Ask your doctor for a simple blood test to know for sure.

Vitamins C and E are anti-oxidant vitamins that may be old school, i.e., boring, at this point in our fad-driven society, but they are still extremely important. Vitamin C has antihistamine properties that can lessen allergic types of inflammation. Vitamin E may reduce activation of mast cells that also play a role in allergies.

Curcumin is an anti-inflammatory natural ingredient in the popular Indian spice tumeric, and it is also available in supplement form. Ayurvedic medicine has traditionally used tumeric for a variety of conditions including arthritis and asthma. Ingesting curcumin eases pain caused by inflammatory diseases of the joints. Better absorbed forms of curcumin may help slow progression of Alzheimer's disease, which involves irreversible damage to brain cells controlling memory.

Magnesium is a mineral that maintains healthy blood pressure and strengthens bones. Magnesium helps to fight against inflammation in the arterial walls. Increasing your magnesium intake can reduce the indicator TNF, which regulates the immune system but can also cause inflammation. The anti-inflammatory properties of this mineral may be one reason why magnesium is linked to a lowered risk of heart disease.

Zinc is a metal that helps to stop the body's immune response. The immune system helps the body to fight off infections, but when the immune response is excessive, you become prone to inflammation. Zinc helps the body to respond to infection appropriately and with less irritation.

Ginger has been used in Ayurvedic medicine to treat arthritis for thousands of years. The anti-inflammatory agents in this root are known as gingerols. Ginger prevents free radicals from damaging lipids in the body. It also suppresses inflammatory compounds in the joints. Joint pain and swelling can drastically reduce when patients ingest ginger daily.

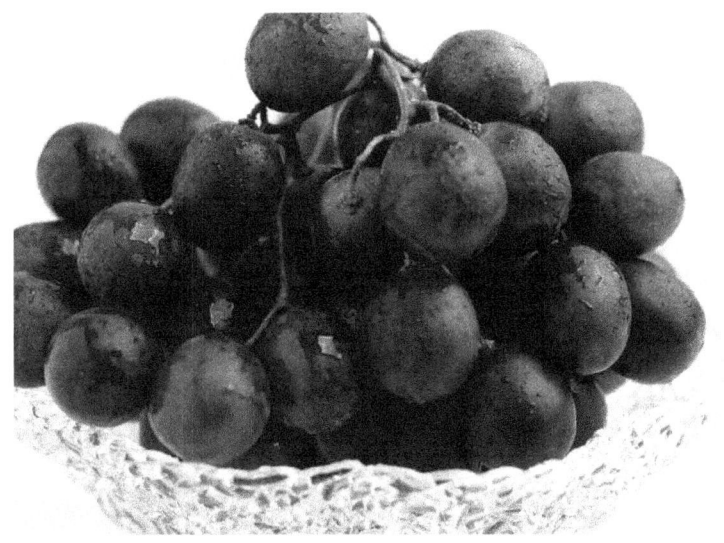

Resveratrol is a plant extract that can be derived from peanuts as well as fruits like grapes. It is frequently used to treat the symptoms of inflammatory bowel disease. Studies show a link between ingestion of resveratrol and suppression of the inflammatory protein TNF-alpha. Resveratrol is also associated with longevity in fruit flies and may promote a longer lifespan in humans.

Alpha-lipoic acid is known as an antioxidant, but it also has powerful properties as an anti-inflammatory agent. It protects nerves from damage by low oxygen levels, free radicals, high blood sugar levels, and even aging. Diabetics with diabetic neuropathy can get drug-free pain relief from alpha-lipoic acid. It may aid bone health by reducing bone loss caused by inflammation. Alpha-lipoic acid may also ease inflammatory symptoms of multiple sclerosis.

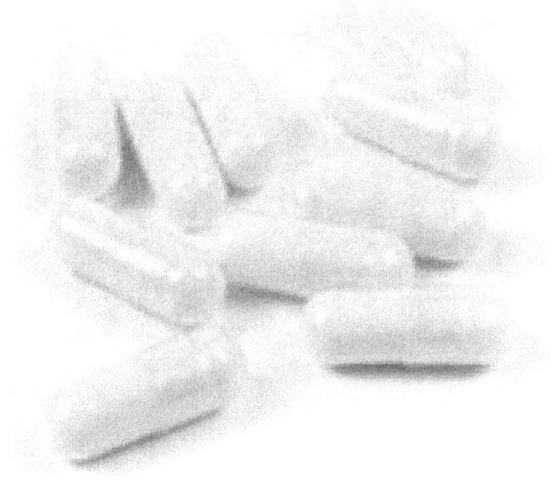

Quercetin is a plant pigment with antioxidant and anti-inflammatory properties. It is especially useful for treating ailments of the heart and blood vessels. Its anti-inflammatory properties can ease pain from fibromyalgia. Quercetin can also reduce oxidative damage to the brain, which means certain highly-bioavailable forms of this plant pigment may help protect against neurodegenerative diseases like Alzheimer's and Parkinson's.

Milk thistle is a flowering herb from the Mediterranean that is best known for promoting health of the liver. The active ingredient in milk thistle, silymarin, heals damage to the cells of the liver. The herb helps reduce liver inflammation as well as supports recovery from hepatitis. Milk thistle is also used to treat inflammation of the gall bladder.

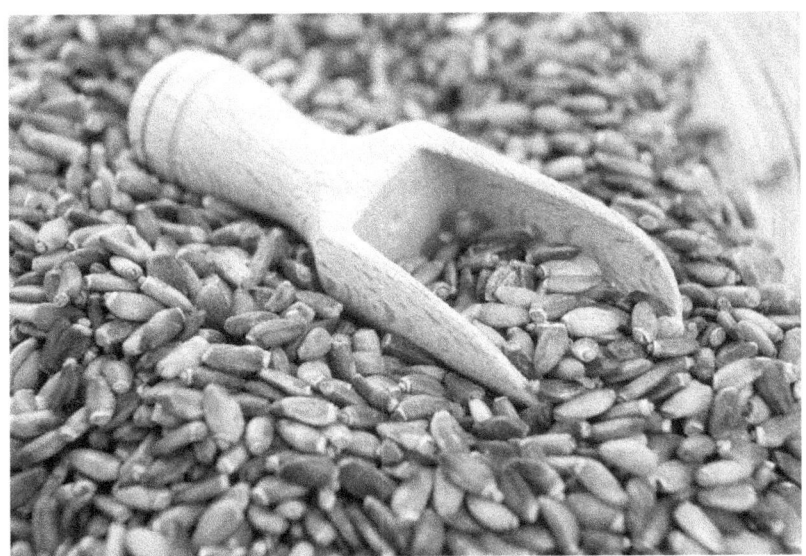

Vitamin K2 is a type of Vitamin K produced by bacteria that is mainly found in the stomach. Vitamin K1 is also beneficial and is involved in blood clotting. K1 can convert to K2 in the body. However, forms of Vitamin K2 have anti-inflammatory properties, and it is best to absorb it directly to get the most of these desirable effects. Vitamin K2 can protect against cardiovascular disease and osteoporosis by reducing inflammation. If you must take an anticoagulant drug like Coumadin or warfarin, discuss this with your doctor before trying any products containing vitamin K.

Probiotics are "good" bacteria that live in your gut. They are supposed to be there. Taking antibiotics or having yeast infections can lead to an overgrowth of bad bacteria that cause poor immune system function throughout your body. Inflammation can result when your intestinal bacteria are not in proper balance. Some studies suggest that certain multi-strain probiotics may lessen the severity of inflammatory bowel disease and Crohn's disease for people with those difficult chronic gastrointestinal inflammatory conditions.

Conclusions

Many of these vitamins and herbs are are a great addition to your daily regimen of vitamins and have few or no side effects. They are easy to find at grocery stores, drug stores or your local health store.

If you are suffering from an inflammatory condition but are concerned about complications from NSAIDs, you may want to supplement your diet with anti-inflammatory herbs and minerals. Then work with your own health care provider to see if it is possible for you to taper and perhaps stop the drugs over time.

Your Action Steps:

1. Find a well-qualified naturopath in your local area to guide you on the individually most helpful nutritional support choices for your personal health problems.

2. **Tell your conventional primary care provider and your pharmacist what you are taking** and ask about possible herb-drug or nutrient-drug interactions that might be a concern for your personal treatment program.

Discuss if you can gradually taper down on pain related drugs like NSAIDs once you have established a good natural anti-inflammatory supplement plan for a while.

3. **Once you have an anti-inflammatory supplement program in place, stick with it.** Nutrients and herbs are slower to act and may need up to 1-3 months to begin to show their beneficial effects. Give them enough time to show you what they can do.

At the same time, other than allergic reactions or herb-drug interactions, side effects of many natural supplements are usually more benign than those of conventional anti-inflammatory drugs, including NSAIDs.

Chapter 6 – Mind-Body Strategies to Reduce Inflammation in the Body

Stress helps promote inflammation in the body. None of us can avoid all stress, but we can change the way we react to our life experiences.

Studies reveal that the mind has an immense ability to impact physical health, both positively and negatively. This is good for those who are struggling with inflammation flare-ups.

You can use your mind for good rather than evil when it comes to your physical body's health. Take some simple steps to offset the effects of stress on your body. If you are a driven person, schedule time-outs for yourself to breathe deeply and use imagery to go to a pleasant nature scene that is calming and peaceful for you.

There have been a number of different non-drug strategies used to help lower inflammation levels in the body, including exercise and diet. Beyond exercise and diet, though, studies have revealed that mind techniques such as meditation and journaling can also reduce stress, potentially lowering the tendency toward chronic inflammation.

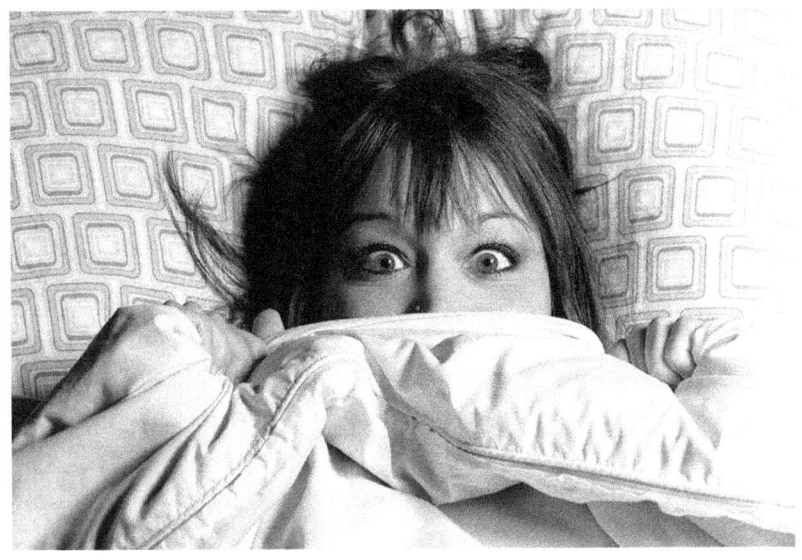

The Role Stress Plays in Causing Inflammation

Physical and emotional stress involves destructive forces within the body that can cause hormone levels to become imbalanced. As a result, stress hormones such as cortisol — which is important for survival — can be released in excess into the bloodstream. This has the potential to alter the body's immune system and even foster increased sensitization to environmental factors.

The effects of chronic stress include a wide range of chronic diseases and complications of existing conditions. People who are stressed caregivers of people with Alzheimer's disease have shortened telomeres, an important structure at the end of chromosomes that carry your genetic information. Shorter telomeres give less protection to the ends of the chromosomes and may increase the aging process along with risks for cancer and death.

Obviously, it appears that you want to protect your telomeres from the ravages of stress. With stress and the perpetual presence of inflammation in the body having negative effects on your health, it is vital to find ways to lower stress and the biological effects it causes in the body.

Anti-Inflammatory Effects of Meditation

Meditation is a type of mind-body practice that involves focused, nonjudgmental attention. Meditation is a component of some Eastern religious and spiritual practices, but there are very accessible types of meditation techniques that have no specific connection with any religion or spiritual belief system.

At its core, meditation involves creating a regular habit of focused quietness, internally and preferably externally. The person practicing medication assumes a relaxed posture or position (but sitting, lying, walking are allowed, depending on the technique). During the process, the goal is openness to experience with an ability to observe but not react emotionally to thoughts that pass through the mind.

In a recent study conducted by researchers in France, Spain and the United States, the researchers were able to draw a clear correlation between meditation and the suppression of the inflammatory signals related to RIPK2 and COX2. Meditation was also able to suppress the histone deactylase gene.

This research provides evidence that people have the power to control expression of their genetic potential with their mind. This is what scientists call epigenetics.

You have the ability to positively influence certain aspects of your physical health through your behavior and thoughts.

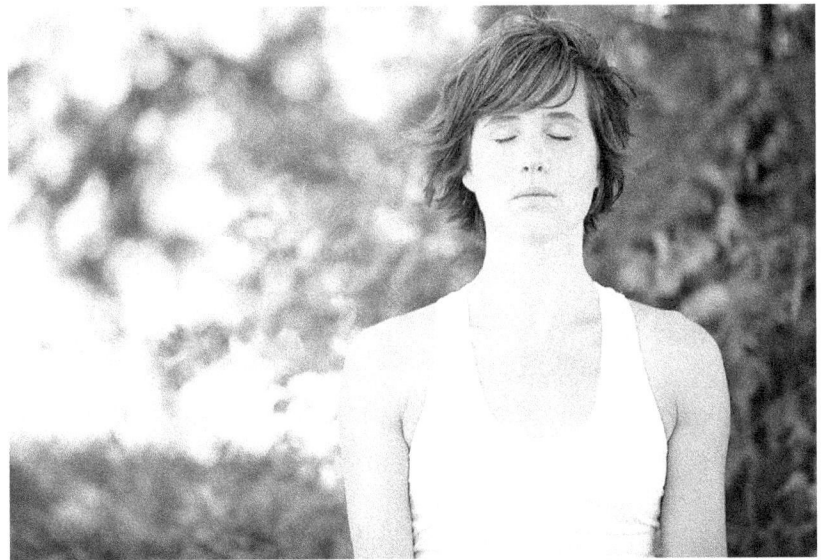

Not only did this study make the connection between the ability of meditation to suppress these genes, but researchers concluded that there is a direct correlation between meditation and the ability to suppress inflammation in the body.

If you are struggling to reduce the level of inflammation in your body, this is good news. The study was actually published in the prestigious journal Psychoneuroendocrinology Journal. In this study subjects showed a significant decrease in pro-inflammatory gene activity after a total of eight hours meditating.

This end result was a faster physical recovery from stress induced physical conditions such as inflammation.

There are many different schools of meditation. Start with one that feels in tune with you, your beliefs, and your health status.

Journaling – More Powerful than You Think

There has been a great deal of data that confirms that humans have the ability to literally think themselves not only sicker, but also, healthier.

Researchers are extremely careful to warn that mind-body approaches are not a substitute for mainstream medicine, but should be used in combination with conventional methods as appropriate to the individual. However there are many natural health experts and physicians who consider meditation as an essential element of good self care.

Writing in a journal, i.e., journaling, may be a simple but effective way to help reduce inflammation. Again, the basic premise is that any lowering of stress levels lower the unhealthy changes that the body undergoes during stress.

It is important to remind yourself that stress is in the eye of the beholder. What bothers you may not bother someone else, or vice versa.

The primary topic for the journaling in research was writing about a stressful experience or situation in a person's life. There are endless studies that have revealed the powerful impact that journaling can have on your ability to elevate your level of creativity, reduce stress, improve the production of positive hormonal and biochemical changes in the body.

A journal is like a best friend forever who will faithfully listen to everything you have to say. It does not interrupt you or give you empty sympathy. It can be direct and even brutally honest. You write your true feelings for you and you alone to read, re-read, meditate on, and grow from. This process is a simple way to un-stifle yourself and say what you really think and feel.

If you have an inflammatory condition such as arthritis or asthma, the evidence suggests that writing in a journal about your stressors may improve your health-related quality of life even months later. This is an incredibly inexpensive and powerful way to improve your health and reduce inflammation. Go for it!

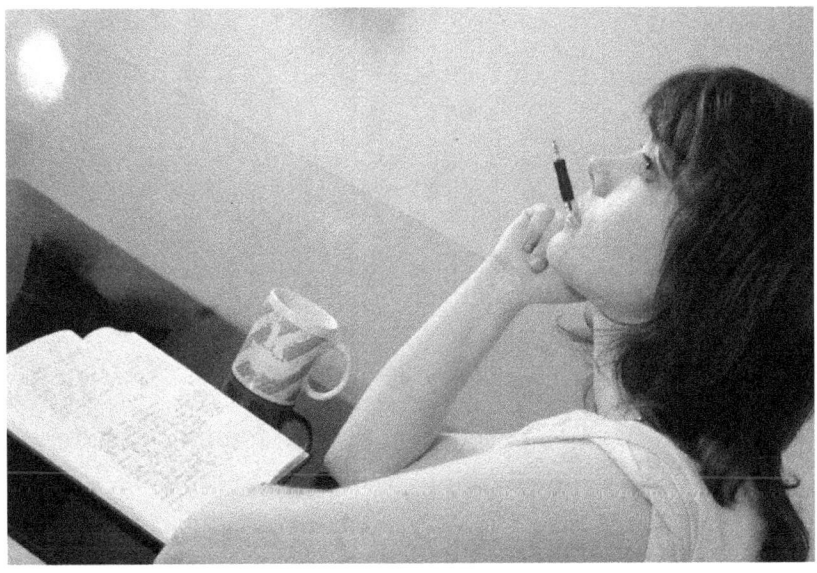

Biofeedback to Reduce Inflammation

Biofeedback is a higher tech type of mind-body technique that focuses on helping patients learn how to use their bodies and minds to control their physiology. Biofeedback helps you learn faster how to regulate heart rate, muscle tension, blood pressure and brainwave frequencies associated with different mental and emotional states. There are both biofeedback professional services available with more advanced equipment and methods and personal biofeedback devices that you can buy online or in stores (visit http://InflammationAdvisor.com/resources to see some options).

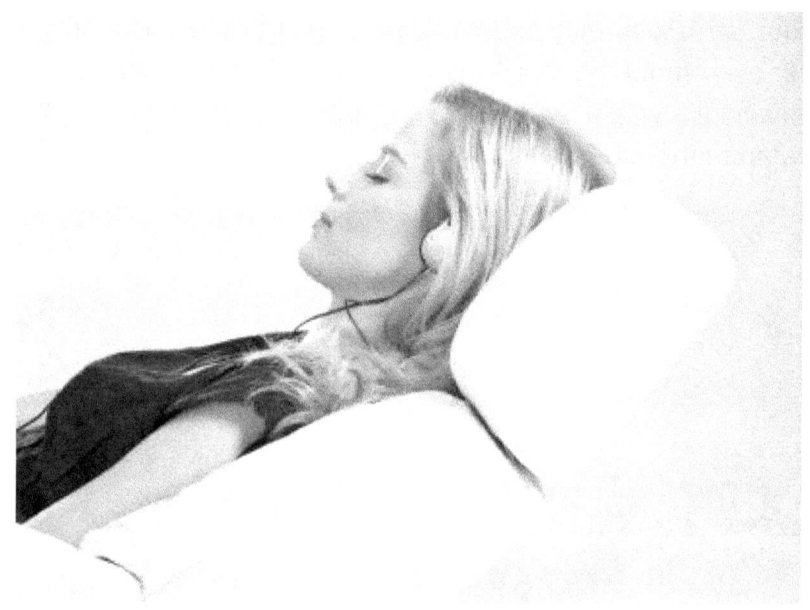

Biofeedback has been used to address a number of different health concerns, including migraines, hypertension, cardiac arrhythmias, stress, anxiety, epilepsy, muscle spasms, chronic pain, inflammation, urinary incontinence, and more. The benefits of biofeedback flow from learning how you are in the moment when your body is producing a healthier way of being as opposed to a less healthy state.

Some biofeedback devices will provide tones or lights, tracings, or video game-like images on a computer screen. These give you moment-to-moment or instantaneous feedback when your state shifts in a "good" or "bad" direction. As you learn to get into the "good" state more of the time, your health benefits.

If you are someone who is never sure if you are doing something like relaxation methods or meditation "correctly," you may find that biofeedback is a valuable tool for you to help yourself faster and with fewer blind alleys. You learn how to allow yourself to be in beneficial states rather than forcing yourself to be in ways that actually cause stress.

If you have read about stress and inflammation at all, you are aware of the significant dangers associated with the persistent presence of chronic inflammation in the body. This is why it is important for you to find some method or methods that are acceptable for you to try.

The mind-body strategies listed here can be used in conjunction with an anti-inflammatory food addiction diet, personal environmental clean-up measures, and any other holistic techniques you include in your program. A multi-pronged approach to reducing inflammation in the body naturally is often more effective than stopping with just one strategy.

With the combination of biofeedback, journaling and regular meditation, you increase your chances of experiencing significant results. But, you don't have to do them all and drive yourself crazy running from "healing" modality to modality. Pick one technique that feels right for you. Explore it. If you enjoy it and it helps, stick with it. Then add others as it seems appropriate until you have maximum benefit.

Guided Imagery

Guided imagery is a mind-body technique that uses words and music to direct and encourage a person to enter into a rich positive state of mind in which the senses and imagination are engaged together.

During imagery, which is similar to self-hypnosis, a person might imagine a peaceful scene for relaxation or recruit white blood cells in the body to fight off an infection or cancer. This mind-body approach can also be very helpful with acute or chronic pain to lessen the need for pain-killing drugs and their unpleasant side effects.

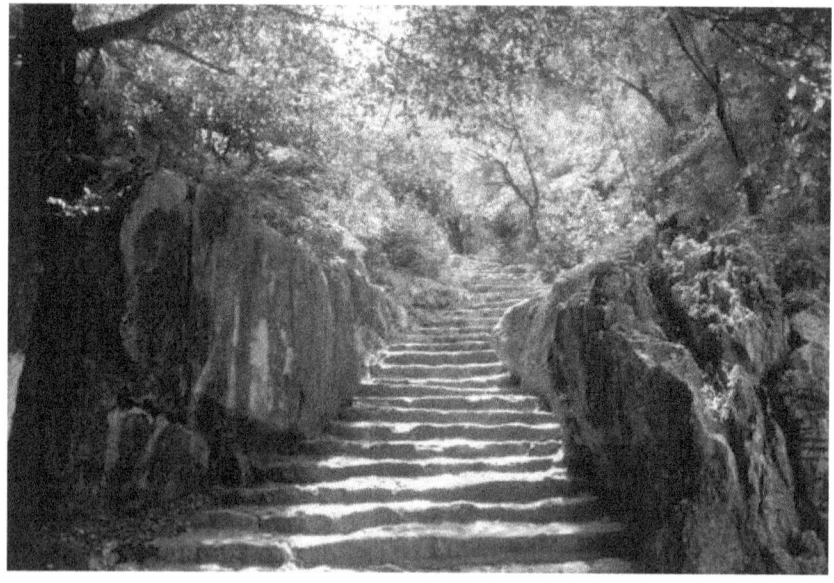

Other types of guided imagery assist people in creating a dialogue with their inner selves to learn answers and insights into their current medical, social, or emotional challenges.

By generating as vivid images as possible in the mind, including sights, sounds, tastes, smells, and touch, you can bypass the conscious mind's defenses that may be keeping you from healing more fully.

Many guided imagery programs are available for self-help in the form of audio downloads or CDs online, some free and some paid. Some audios are available free. At the time of this writing, here are only a few of many examples:

- Dartmouth Health Promotion and Wellness Program - http://www.dartmouth.edu/~healthed/relax/downloads.html

- Inner Health Studio - http://www.innerhealthstudio.com/guided-imagery.html

- Health Journeys - http://www.healthjourneys.com/free_audio.asp

- Guided Imagery Downloads - http://www.guidedimagerydownloads.com/

Some guided imagery programs from experienced practitioners would include, but are not limited to:

- The Healing Mind – http://thehealingmind.org

- Academy of Guided Imagery - http://acadgi.com/index.html

- Cleveland Clinic Guided Imagery Services in the Integrative Medicine Division - http://my.clevelandclinic.org/wellness/integrative-medicine/treatments-services/guided-imagery.aspx

- Kaiser-Permanente Healthcare – https://healthy.kaiserpermanente.org/health/care/!u t/p/a0/FchBDoMgEADAt_iAzYZEYfFmhH6hhdsGiZIIG ELt99seZ9DjC33hO- 3cUy18_uxCLD22md9bqnCnLVZ8okd_Nd4zoysVAocj_ o9bT- GM6IzVap2MBamlBCGsgEWPBohoUkKp8UErXjnTZx mGL2IKPpI!/

Obviously, since you want to be able to let your mind go into a relaxed altered state for guided imagery, often with your eyes closed, you should not listen to these types of programs while driving or operating dangerous machinery or equipment.

Your Action Steps:

1. **Get a good practical summary of stress reduction and relaxation methods** such as the classic book, *The Relaxation and Stress Reduction Workbook.* You can find it available online or in bookstores.

2. **Choose at least one and perhaps two mind-body techniques for healing** that fit in with who you are and how you can add these as a new daily habit to support your inflammatory health.

3. **Obtain the audios, videos, books, and/or devices** you need to implement your chosen mind-body techniques daily in the comfort of your own home.

4. **Schedule your mind-body therapy times daily** (e.g., 15-20 minutes per day) and treat these times as appointments with an important client – yourself. You are your strongest advocate for healing and heath care provider.

Chapter 7 – Holistic Therapies for Reducing Inflammation Naturally

In dealing with inflammatory diseases from IBD (Inflammatory Bowel Disease) to rheumatoid arthritis, you want to know about as broad a set of options for drug-free treatments as possible.

Holistic is a general term for types of health care that (a) take the whole person into consideration at once, rather than body part by body parts; and (b) rely on interventions that use diagnostic and treatment methods to rebalance or set right the person as a whole system or interconnected network.

What are the best treatments? Are the practitioners well-trained and credentialed? How much will the treatments cost? Will the treatment "cure," cause side effects, or simply alleviate discomfort? These are all valid questions to ask potential practitioners as you explore your options.

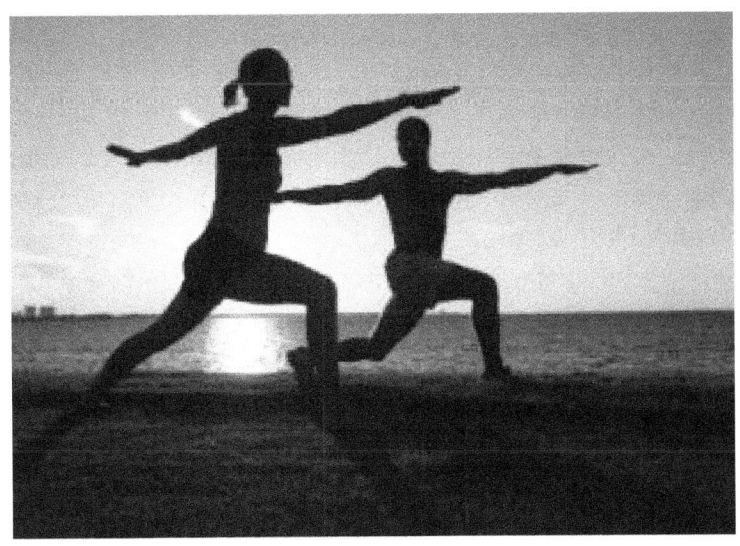

Sacrificing your health should not have to be an option. In addition to the mind-body approaches discussed in the previous chapter, other holistic treatments like Tai Chi, qigong, acupuncture and homeopathy offer promising results. The term "holistic" is not some fancy method that only elite spas and expensive hotels use.

Holistic treatments and therapies for inflammatory diseases are usually intended to address root disturbances in the person as an integrated being or complex adaptive system. The whole is greater than the sum of the parts. Your environment is in constant flux – which causes your body (and mind) to adjust constantly as well.

Being adaptive and resilient in the face of changes in your internal and external environment is a sign of good health. But sometimes you run out of reserves and disease develops when the environmental changes overwhelm you. Chronic stress is one factor in overwhelming reserves and adaptation.

In holistic approaches, instead of treating the symptoms at a superficial level by suppressing the wheezing with a drug inhaler, holistic treatments would invite the entire body to get on board with the healing process.

There are many misunderstandings about how our bodies operate on a day-to-day basis, much less when fighting for its survival. The bottom line of healthful treatment is to understand your body is a system, an eco-system, if you will. When one element is either positively or negatively affected, the functioning of interconnected elements is also affected, creating a domino effect throughout the body.

It is important to make sure cellular conversations in the body are friendly, supportive and encouraging. Otherwise, some of the neighbors will start to complain. Even worse, some of the more protective neighboring cells may take matters into their own molecular hands by turning on the floodgates of mediators that produce inflammation, pain, fluid, and disease. Then, here comes the inflammation.

This disciplinary or regulatory reaction is basic and often oddly beneficial. But in the long run, any type of flood can damage and may even kill. Long story short, your body doesn't appreciate too much inflammation for long periods of time. Several different holistic therapies can get your parts talking in better harmony with one another.

Acupuncture

Acupuncture is an Eastern medical art treatment with millennia of tradition behind it. When small needles are inserted into the skin in precise locations, specific unique locations are targeted for the purpose of signaling your body to rebalance its energetic flow and heal.

Acupuncture is a part of the larger whole system of traditional Chinese medicine, which also includes diet, complex herbal formulas, qi gong as exercise, and a type of massage called tui na.

Furthermore, there are a number of other styles and schools of thought in this field. The overall treatment goal is to understand the symptoms as manifestations of energetic excesses, deficiencies, relative imbalances and blockages across the person as a unified being.

In Chinese medicine theory, the person is a network of meridian channels and hubs or acupoints representing different subsystems and their interrelationships. The body contains various microcosms of the larger environment within it.

In the modern era, some acupuncture experts have developed ways of stimulating or sedating acupuncture points without needles, i.e., using laser light or electromagnetic signals. There are also Korean and Japanese styles of acupuncture, as well as Western forms of medical acupuncture.

A recent article titled "Acupuncture Holds Promise for Treating Inflammatory Disease," from Rutgers University in New Jersey, electroacupuncture treatments on mice was for a

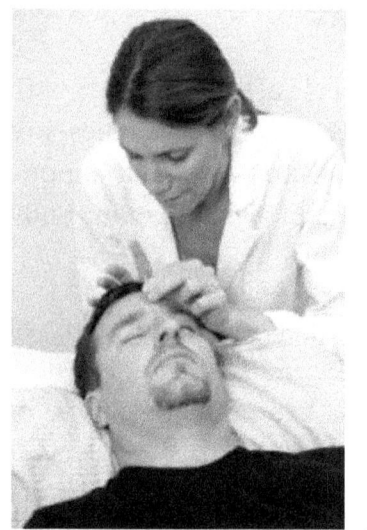

specific and often deadly inflammatory condition called "sepsis." Sepsis occurs as a life-threatening consequence of a serious infection in which an infection goes out of control. The sepsis occurs in response to overwhelming bacteria and bacterial toxins released into the body. Blood pressure can fall to dangerously low levels and multiple organs fail.

With nerve stimulation using electroacupuncture, the sepsis study showed a positive effect of stimulation on dopamine and cytokine molecular levels, two of the body's molecular mediators and regulators of inflammatory and immune system responses.

In more usual outpatient care, acupuncture is reported to be helpful for health problems that range from arthritis to headache to chemotherapy-related nausea and vomiting. As discussed earlier, certain acupuncture treatments may lessen addictive cravings and help an addicted person get through withdrawal symptoms.

Getting your body to respond naturally, without chemicals is a smart beginning. Overall, acupuncture is a historically safe and beneficial way to re-regulate how the body functions as an intact or integrated living system. You can find a local acupuncturist at http://Acufinder.com and compare their qualifications and approach to treatment.

Homeopathy

Homeopathy is an over 200-year-old system of alternative medicine founded by a German physician and chemist named Samuel Hahnemann, MD. Homeopathy uses small doses of medicines prepared in a special manner from natural plant, mineral, or animal sources.

The preparation process includes long periods of intensive grinding of insoluble materials in milk sugar or lactose and/or serial dilutions and successions (multiple powerful strokes or agitations of the glassware containing the source material in a water or an ethanol-water solution.

Recent studies demonstrate that these preparation methods generate tiny, albeit crude, forms of particles from source material and silica from the inside walls of the glass. It is now easy to find nanotechnology papers in the drug delivery research literature that describe how prolonged milling of insoluble materials in dry or wet media will make smaller and smaller, more biologically available and effective nanoparticles of source material. These nanoparticles can have unique enhanced biological effects at low doses.

Homeopaths have scientific evidence to support the ability of the manufacturing methods to generate smaller particles and biologically active medicines that affect cells, plants, animals, and human beings. Although skeptics often claim that homeopathic medicines are only inert placebos, many, though not all, studies show properties and effects different from those of placebo controls.

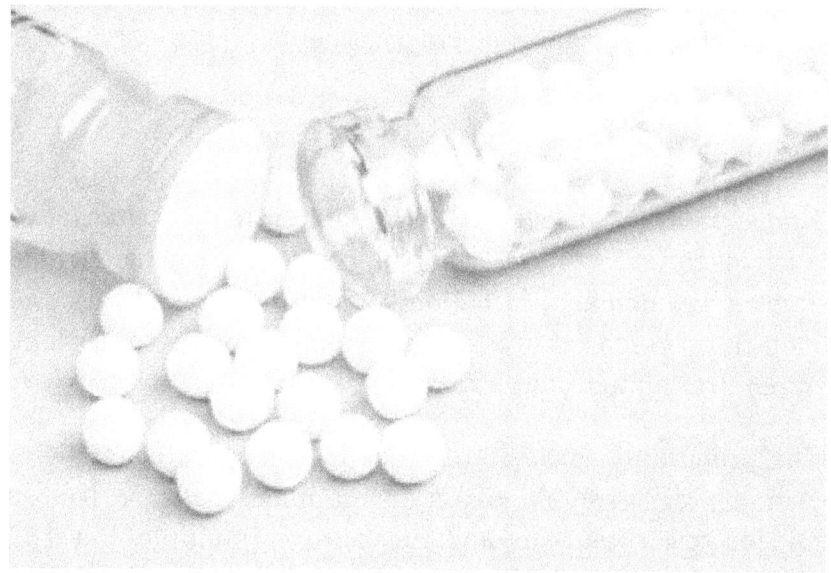

Like acupuncturists, homeopaths view the person as an integrated living system in which a unified treatment that properly addresses the complete biopsychosocial symptom picture of the individual can initiate a person-wide healing process. Homeopaths often treat health problems involving inflammation such as allergies, fibromyalgia, and various autoimmune diseases.

In general, homeopaths, like acupuncturists, treat the person constitutionally, that is, as a whole system, not as a conventionally-diagnosed medical condition in an isolated body part. However, in acute injuries and illnesses, it is sometimes possible to use only a small handful of homeopathic medicines for a given acute problem. Some studies suggest that homeopathically prepared substances such as Apis from the honey bee may help produce less fluid accumulation and swelling in affected individuals.

For example, one recent study showed that homeopathic Apis can modify the expression of hundreds or different genes at once. Low versus high dilutions can produce effects in opposite directions. This is one of several test tube studies suggesting that homeopathic medicines may act as epigenetic modulators or modifiers of gene expression. By turning specific genes on and off, the cells end up making different proteins and signaling cells of the body in complex ways.

For self-care, there are some combination homeopathic medicines available that include a number of different individual ingredients to cover what a majority of people with a given acute problem may experience in symptom patterns.

However, a typical homeopath will take a careful history and prescribe only one medicine at a time to treat the total picture of symptoms that the specific person reports. To learn more about homeopathy or find a practitioner, visit the website of the National Center for Homeopathy (http://homeopathycenter.org).

For a chronic inflammatory illness, it is highly preferable to consult a well-qualified practitioner and not to try to treat yourself with homeopathy for the long term.

Tai Chi and Qigong as Therapy

Here is an ancient traditional self care technique from Chinese medicine - Tai Chi for inflammation. If you are like the rest of us, you are willing to explore everything available to help reduce the drudgeries of inflammatory issues.

Tai Chi or T'ai chi ch'uan, an internal Chinese martial art form, can work wonders for inflammation by reorganizing our body's systemic energies and natural energy flow to improve our natural healing processes. This addition to daily self-care health maintenance and treatment routines has a positive reputation for success in improving quality of life.

Tai chi and another traditional Chinese healing method, qi gong, for medical purposes have enjoyed a respected place in self-care for thousands of years. Older folks may especially benefit from the gentle, graceful, slow movements and positions involved.

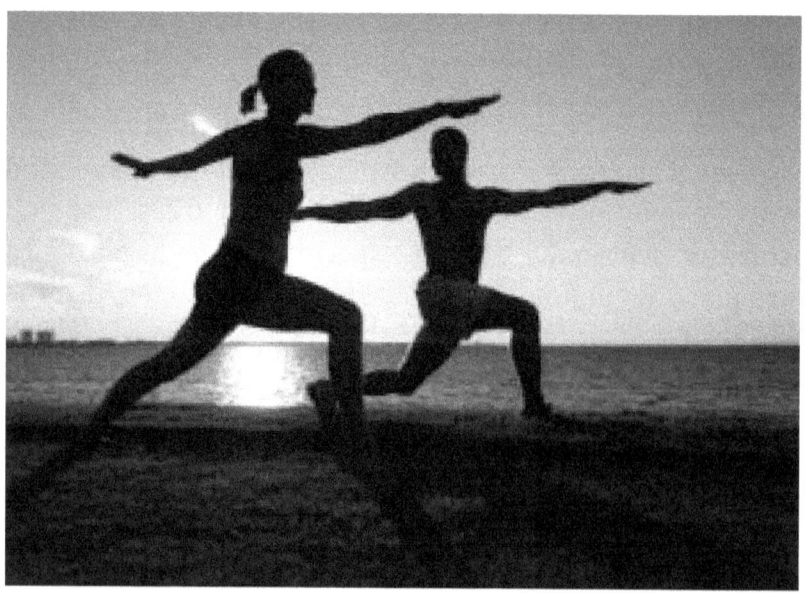

It is typically best to learn from an experienced teacher who knows who to adapt the specific positions and techniques for individual health challenges. Along with the mind-body methods discussed elsewhere in this book, tai chi and qi gong offer a way to improve balance and lower stress. An obvious benefit is to reduce the biology of inflammation and its associated pain and physical discomforts.

Another powerful energy medicine component of traditional Chinese medicine is qigong. Qigong or qi gong is an ancient healing method for self care and for practitioner-provided healing.

There are also many different schools of qi gong available. One very accessible type that is focused on helping people recover from chronic illness through self-healing is Spring Forest Qigong. You can learn more about it at http://www.springforestqigong.com/.

Conclusion

Using holistic therapies for inflammatory diseases, even when integrated with conventional medical practices, not only enhances the natural course of healing, they also offer a reminder of the natural powers for healing in your own body and mind.

Your inflammation and the diseases associated with it do not define you. Get the help you need with holistic measures to define the life you love and to live it - your way.

Your Action Steps:

1. To support your whole person healing, **choose either acupuncture or homeopathy** as constitutional treatment towards healing the inflammation processes in your body. Find a practitioner using the resources listed above.

2. **Find out more about tai chi or qigong classes in your area** or get an introductory audio/CD/DVD program to learn about the area to help you with your personal health challenges.

3. **Add regular tai chi or qigong practice** to support and enhance your healing and health.

Next Steps

This book provides you an introduction to the nature of inflammation and natural, drug-free ways to find help for chronic health problems associated with inflammatory mechanisms.

One of the goals has been to arm you as the informed consumer with an awareness of how many different types of treatment can be focused on reducing inflammation in the body and improving your quality of life.

It is now up to you to decide what to do next. You have action steps in each chapter. If you need more help, learn more about our step-by-step modular online educational program for people with inflammatory conditions. You can find it at http://ReducingInflammationNaturally.com.

Don't forget to check out our free bonus download offer at the end of this book as well. Keep in touch with us at http://InflammationAdvisor.com. We update our Resources page and post news and commentary on developments in the field regularly.

If you want more for yourself than drugs, keep learning and keep trying. You want to be thoughtful and rational in your choices,

As the well-known quotation from the philosopher Lao Tzu says, *"The journey of a thousand miles begins with one step."* For your own good, make the choice now to take that first step.

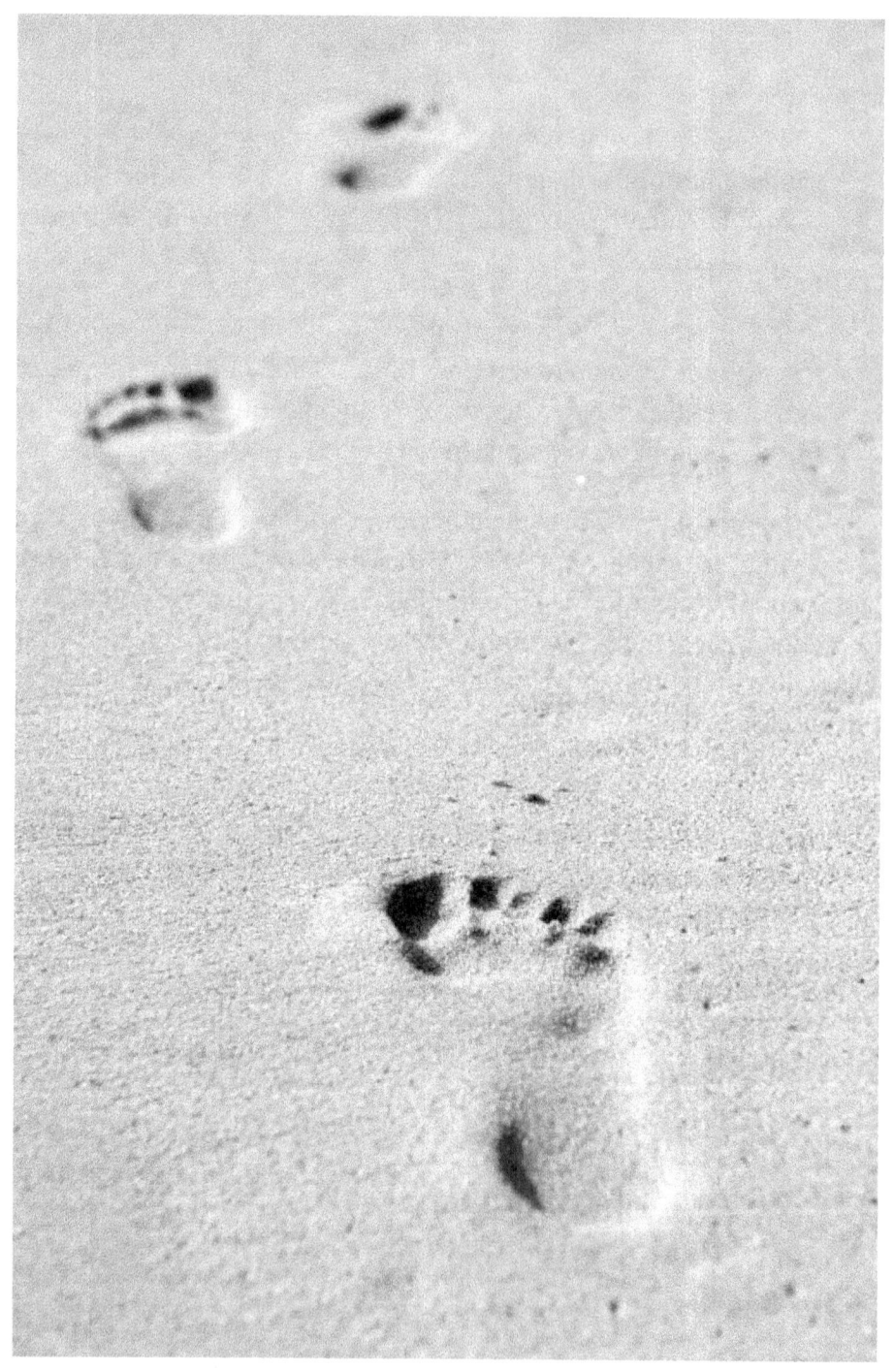

Resources

Find a local naturopath

http://www.naturopathic.org/AF_MemberDirectory.asp?version=2

Find a local acupuncturist

http://acufinder.com or
http://www.thirdage.com/d/dr/spc-1/acupuncturists

Find a local homeopath

http://www.homeopathycenter.org/

Learn about Spring Forest Qigong healing

http://www.springforestqigong.com/

For many additional options, visit our updated Resources page at

http://inflammationadvisor.com/resources/

About the Author

Iris R. Bell, MD, PhD, is a Board-certified psychiatrist and university professor emeritus. As a past member of the academic faculties at the University of California -- San Francisco, Harvard Medical School, and the University of Arizona College of Medicine, she wrote scores of professional research papers on topics ranging from psychiatry to biofeedback and alternative medicine. Her current focus is to help people with chronic inflammatory health issues find drug-free natural self-care solutions to improve their quality of life. She consults, teaches, writes, and lives in Tucson, Arizona with her two dogs, Rocky and Annie.

Thank You -- Bonus Offer!

If you enjoyed this book, would you please take a moment to leave a review on Amazon? Short or long, it may help other people who are also looking for natural self help approaches to support their own health.

To leave a review, visit
http://InflammationAdvisor.com/inflammation-101-review

"Who Else Wants A Special Anti Inflammatory Living Resource List, Checklist and Bonus Recipes...?"

Claim Your FREE Printable Copy of the *Inflammation Advisor's* Quick Start Anti Inflammatory Living Resource List, Checklist, Bonus Anti Inflammatory Recipes, Expanded Resource List, Updates and More...

Claim Your FREE BONUS at
http://InflammationAdvisor.com/inflammation-101-bonus

Ready for More In-Depth Help?

Discover the step by step secrets of reducing inflammation naturally with our complete self-paced 4-module program. Here you will find the how-to details with which you can put these ideas into action. Build upon the information in this book and go way beyond to empowering yourself for informed self care...

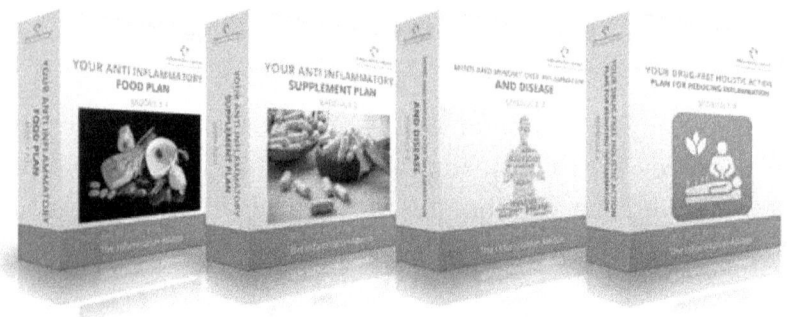

Check out The Inflammation Advisor's "Fight Inflammatory Disease Naturally – Your Complete Drug Free Strategic Program" at http://ReducingInflammationNaturally.com

www.ingramcontent.com/pod-product-compliance
Lightning Source LLC
Chambersburg PA
CBHW071617170526
45166CB00003B/1100